APHASIA COOKBOOK

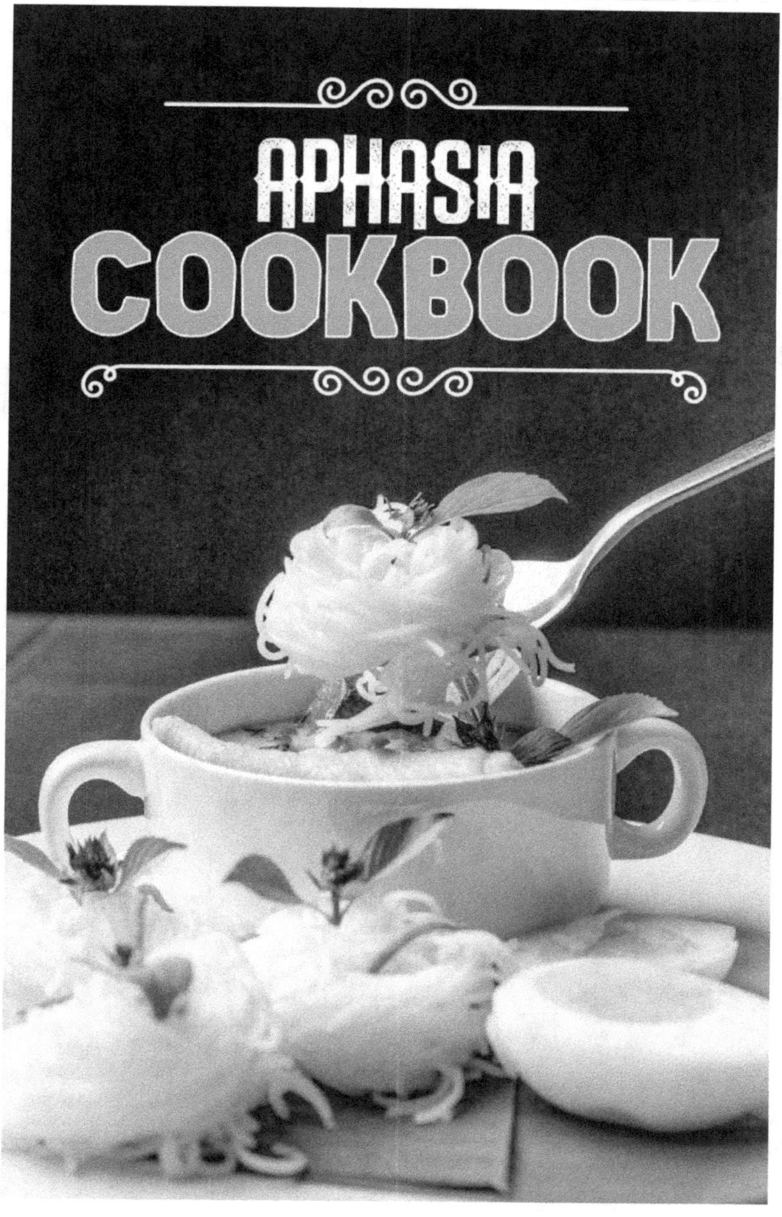

This book belongs to...

Aphasia Cookbook

Recipes to Nourish and Boost Health

-- Drusilla Ronnell Allison --

Attribution

This cover was designed with help from pexels.com

ISBN

9798323351466

Imprint

Independently Published

== Disclaimer ==

The information contained in this book is for general informational purposes only. The author and publisher have made every effort to ensure that the content provided is accurate and up-to-date at the time of publication. However, medical knowledge is constantly evolving, and individual circumstances vary. Therefore, the author and publisher do not make any representations or warranties of any kind, express or implied, about the completeness, accuracy, reliability, suitability, or availability of the information contained in this book.

The information provided is not a substitute for professional medical advice, diagnosis, or treatment. Always seek the advice of your physician or another qualified healthcare provider with any questions you may have regarding a medical condition. Never disregard professional medical advice or delay seeking it because of something you have read in this book.

The author and publisher disclaim any responsibility for any adverse effects resulting directly or indirectly from the use of the information provided in this book. The reader assumes full responsibility for consulting a qualified healthcare professional regarding health conditions and before starting any new treatment or making changes to existing treatment.

The inclusion of specific products, services, or medical procedures in this book does not imply endorsement. The author and publisher shall have no liability for any damages or loss arising out of, or in connection with, the use of this book.

It is recommended to independently verify any information provided in this book and consult with a qualified healthcare professional for advice tailored to your individual circumstances.

List of Contents

Personal Note for This Cookbook

As you flip through the pages of this cookbook, I hope you find not just recipes, but moments of comfort, joy, and nourishment. Creating this collection has been a labor of love, inspired by the journey of those facing aphasia and their caregivers.

Food has a unique power to bring people together, to soothe the soul, and to nourish the body. It is my sincere hope that the recipes contained within these pages serve as more than just instructions; may they be a source of connection, resilience, and healing.

To those navigating the challenges of aphasia, know that you are not alone. Whether it's a warm bowl of soup on a chilly day or a slice of homemade bread shared with loved ones, may these recipes offer moments of solace and strength.

Important note about this book: Please note that the information provided here is for general knowledge and should not replace professional medical advice. If you have specific concerns or questions about **Aphasia**, it's best to consult with a healthcare professional familiar with your medical history.

1. Introduction

Welcome to the Aphasia Cookbook, a collection of recipes crafted with care and consideration for those navigating the journey of aphasia. Aphasia, a condition that affects one's ability to communicate, can present unique challenges in everyday life. From difficulty finding the right words to struggles with reading and writing, aphasia touches every aspect of daily living.

In the face of these challenges, food can serve as a source of comfort, connection, and nourishment. This cookbook is more than just a compilation of recipes; it's a testament to the resilience and creativity of individuals living with aphasia and their caregivers. Each recipe has been thoughtfully curated to provide delicious and nutritious options that are both accessible and enjoyable.

Whether you're seeking simple meals for busy days, comforting dishes for moments of solace, or innovative ideas to spark conversation, the Aphasia Cookbook has something for everyone. From hearty soups and satisfying salads to flavorful entrees and delightful desserts, these recipes aim to inspire and delight the senses.

As you embark on this culinary journey, remember that you are not alone. May these recipes bring joy to your kitchen, warmth to your table, and moments of connection with loved ones. Together, let's savor the simple pleasures of food and the power it holds to nourish both body and soul.

2. **Hearty Vegetable Soup**

Ingredients:

- 2 tablespoons olive oil
- 1 onion, chopped
- 2 cloves garlic, minced
- 3 carrots, diced
- 2 celery stalks, diced
- 1 bell pepper, diced
- 1 zucchini, diced
- 1 can diced tomatoes
- 4 cups vegetable broth
- 1 teaspoon dried thyme
- Salt and pepper to taste
- Fresh parsley for garnish

Instructions:

1. In a large pot, heat olive oil over medium heat. Add onion and garlic, sauté until translucent.

2. Add carrots, celery, bell pepper, and zucchini. Cook for 5 minutes, stirring occasionally.

3. Pour in diced tomatoes and vegetable broth. Add thyme, salt, and pepper. Bring to a boil, then reduce heat and let simmer for 20-25 minutes.

4. Once vegetables are tender, taste and adjust seasoning if needed. Serve hot, garnished with fresh parsley.

3. Quinoa Salad with Lemon-Herb Dressing

Ingredients:

- 1 cup quinoa, rinsed
- 2 cups water
- 1 cucumber, diced
- 1 cup cherry tomatoes, halved
- 1/4 cup red onion, finely chopped
- 1/4 cup fresh parsley, chopped
- 1/4 cup fresh mint, chopped
- Juice of 1 lemon
- 2 tablespoons olive oil
- Salt and pepper to taste

Instructions:

1. In a medium saucepan, bring water to a boil. Add quinoa, reduce heat to low, cover, and simmer for 15 minutes or until water is absorbed. Remove from heat and let cool.

2. In a large bowl, combine cooked quinoa, cucumber, cherry tomatoes, red onion, parsley, and mint.

3. In a small bowl, whisk together lemon juice, olive oil, salt, and pepper to make the dressing.

4. Pour dressing over the salad and toss to combine. Adjust seasoning if needed. Serve chilled or at room temperature.

4. Baked Salmon with Roasted Vegetables

Ingredients:

- 4 salmon fillets
- 2 tablespoons olive oil
- 1 tablespoon lemon juice
- 2 cloves garlic, minced
- 1 teaspoon dried thyme
- Salt and pepper to taste
- 2 cups mixed vegetables (such as broccoli, bell peppers, and carrots), chopped

Instructions:

1. Preheat oven to 400°F (200°C). Line a baking sheet with parchment paper.
2. In a small bowl, whisk together olive oil, lemon juice, garlic, thyme, salt, and pepper.
3. Place salmon fillets on the prepared baking sheet. Brush with the olive oil mixture.

4. In a separate bowl, toss mixed vegetables with remaining olive oil mixture. Spread them around the salmon on the baking sheet.

5. Bake for 15-20 minutes, or until salmon is cooked through and vegetables are tender. Serve hot.

5. Spinach and Mushroom Omelette

Ingredients:

- 4 large eggs

- 1/4 cup milk

- Salt and pepper to taste

- 1 tablespoon butter

- 1 cup baby spinach leaves

- 1/2 cup sliced mushrooms

- 1/4 cup shredded cheese (such as cheddar or feta)

Instructions:

1. In a bowl, whisk together eggs, milk, salt, and pepper until well combined.

2. In a non-stick skillet, melt butter over medium heat. Add spinach and mushrooms, sauté until spinach is wilted and mushrooms are tender.

3. Pour the egg mixture over the spinach and mushrooms in the skillet. Cook for 2-3 minutes,

lifting the edges with a spatula to let the uncooked egg flow underneath.

4. Sprinkle shredded cheese over one half of the omelette. Fold the other half over the cheese. Cook for another minute until cheese is melted and the omelette is cooked through.

5. Slide the omelette onto a plate and serve hot.

6. Banana-Oat Breakfast Smoothie

Ingredients:

- 1 ripe banana
- 1/2 cup rolled oats
- 1/2 cup Greek yogurt
- 1/2 cup milk (or dairy-free alternative)
- 1 tablespoon honey (optional)
- 1/2 teaspoon vanilla extract
- Pinch of cinnamon

Instructions:

1. Place all ingredients in a blender.

2. Blend until smooth and creamy, adding more milk if necessary to reach desired consistency.

3. Taste and adjust sweetness with honey if desired.

4. Pour into glasses and serve immediately.

7. Turkey and Veggie Stir-Fry

Ingredients:

- 1 tablespoon vegetable oil
- 1 pound turkey breast, sliced into thin strips
- 2 cups mixed vegetables (such as bell peppers, broccoli, carrots, and snap peas), sliced
- 3 cloves garlic, minced
- 2 tablespoons soy sauce
- 1 tablespoon hoisin sauce
- 1 teaspoon sesame oil
- Cooked rice or noodles, for serving

Instructions:

1. Heat vegetable oil in a large skillet or wok over high heat.

2. Add turkey strips and cook until browned and cooked through, about 5-6 minutes. Remove from skillet and set aside.

3. In the same skillet, add mixed vegetables and garlic. Stir-fry for 3-4 minutes until vegetables are tender-crisp.

4. Return cooked turkey to the skillet. Add soy sauce, hoisin sauce, and sesame oil. Stir-fry for another 2 minutes to combine flavors.

5. Serve hot over cooked rice or noodles.

8. Sweet Potato and Black Bean Chili

Ingredients:

- 2 tablespoons olive oil
- 1 onion, diced
- 2 cloves garlic, minced
- 1 sweet potato, peeled and diced
- 1 bell pepper, diced
- 1 can black beans, drained and rinsed
- 1 can diced tomatoes
- 2 cups vegetable broth
- 2 teaspoons chili powder
- 1 teaspoon ground cumin
- Salt and pepper to taste

- Optional toppings: chopped cilantro, avocado slices, shredded cheese, sour cream

Instructions:

1. Heat olive oil in a large pot over medium heat. Add onion and garlic, sauté until softened.

2. Add sweet potato and bell pepper, cook for 5 minutes.

3. Stir in black beans, diced tomatoes, vegetable broth, chili powder, cumin, salt, and pepper.

4. Bring to a boil, then reduce heat and let simmer for 20-25 minutes, until sweet potatoes are tender and flavors are well combined.

5. Serve hot, topped with optional toppings if desired.

9. Greek Yogurt Parfait with Berries and Granola

Ingredients:

- 1 cup Greek yogurt

- 1/2 cup mixed berries (such as strawberries, blueberries, raspberries)

- 1/4 cup granola

- 1 tablespoon honey (optional)

Instructions:

1. In a serving glass or bowl, layer Greek yogurt, mixed berries, and granola.

2. Drizzle honey on top if desired.

3. Repeat layers if using a larger serving container.

4. Serve immediately as a nutritious breakfast or snack.

10.Chicken and Vegetable Quinoa Bowl

Ingredients:

- 1 cup quinoa, rinsed

- 2 cups water or chicken broth

- 1 tablespoon olive oil

- 2 boneless, skinless chicken breasts, diced

- 2 cups mixed vegetables (such as bell peppers, broccoli, carrots)

- Salt and pepper to taste

- 2 tablespoons soy sauce

- 1 tablespoon honey

- 1 teaspoon sesame oil

- Sesame seeds for garnish (optional)

Instructions:

1. In a medium saucepan, bring water or chicken broth to a boil. Add quinoa, reduce heat to low, cover, and simmer for 15 minutes or until liquid is absorbed. Fluff with a fork and set aside.

2. In a large skillet, heat olive oil over medium-high heat. Add diced chicken and cook until browned and cooked through, about 5-6 minutes. Remove from skillet and set aside.

3. In the same skillet, add mixed vegetables and cook until tender-crisp, about 3-4 minutes.

4. Return cooked chicken to the skillet. Add soy sauce, honey, and sesame oil. Stir to combine and heat through.

5. To serve, divide quinoa among bowls, top with chicken and vegetable mixture. Garnish with sesame seeds if desired.

11.Mango and Avocado Salad

Ingredients:

- 2 ripe mangoes, peeled and diced
- 1 ripe avocado, peeled, pitted, and diced
- 1/4 cup red onion, finely chopped
- 1/4 cup fresh cilantro, chopped
- Juice of 1 lime
- Salt and pepper to taste
- Optional: diced jalapeño for a spicy kick

Instructions:

1. In a large bowl, combine diced mangoes, avocado, red onion, and cilantro.
2. Squeeze lime juice over the salad and toss gently to combine.
3. Season with salt and pepper to taste.
4. If desired, add diced jalapeño for extra heat.
5. Serve immediately as a refreshing side dish or light lunch.

12. Turkey and Vegetable Meatball Soup

Ingredients:

- 1 pound ground turkey
- 1/4 cup breadcrumbs
- 1 egg
- 1/4 cup grated Parmesan cheese
- 1/4 cup finely chopped onion
- 2 cloves garlic, minced
- 1 teaspoon dried oregano
- 1 teaspoon dried basil
- Salt and pepper to taste
- 8 cups chicken broth
- 2 carrots, diced
- 2 celery stalks, diced
- 1 cup small pasta (such as ditalini or orzo)
- Fresh parsley for garnish

Instructions:

1. In a large bowl, combine ground turkey, breadcrumbs, egg, Parmesan cheese, onion, garlic, oregano, basil, salt, and pepper. Mix until well combined.

2. Shape the mixture into small meatballs, about 1 inch in diameter.

3. In a large pot, bring chicken broth to a simmer over medium heat. Add carrots, celery, and pasta. Cook for 8-10 minutes until pasta is tender.

4. Gently drop the meatballs into the simmering broth. Cook for another 8-10 minutes until meatballs are cooked through.

5. Taste and adjust seasoning if needed. Serve hot, garnished with fresh parsley.

13.Coconut Curry Lentil Soup

Ingredients:

- 1 tablespoon coconut oil

- 1 onion, diced

- 2 cloves garlic, minced

- 1 tablespoon grated ginger

- 1 tablespoon curry powder

- 1 cup dried red lentils, rinsed

- 4 cups vegetable broth

- 1 can (14 ounces) coconut milk

- 2 cups chopped spinach or kale

- Juice of 1 lime

- Salt and pepper to taste

Instructions:

1. In a large pot, heat coconut oil over medium heat. Add onion, garlic, and ginger. Sauté until softened and fragrant.

2. Stir in curry powder and cook for another minute.

3. Add red lentils and vegetable broth. Bring to a boil, then reduce heat and let simmer for 15-20 minutes until lentils are tender.

4. Stir in coconut milk and chopped spinach or kale. Simmer for another 5 minutes until greens are wilted.

5. Stir in lime juice and season with salt and pepper to taste.

6. Serve hot as a comforting and flavorful soup option.

14. Roasted Vegetable and Quinoa Salad

Ingredients:

- 1 cup quinoa, rinsed

- 2 cups water or vegetable broth

- 2 cups mixed vegetables (such as bell peppers, zucchini, cherry tomatoes, red onion), chopped

- 2 tablespoons olive oil

- 1 teaspoon dried herbs (such as thyme, rosemary, or oregano)

- Salt and pepper to taste

- 1/4 cup crumbled feta cheese (optional)

- Balsamic glaze for drizzling (optional)

Instructions:

1. Preheat the oven to 400°F (200°C).

2. In a medium saucepan, bring water or vegetable broth to a boil. Add quinoa, reduce heat to low, cover, and simmer for 15 minutes or until liquid is absorbed. Fluff with a fork and set aside.

3. Place chopped vegetables on a baking sheet. Drizzle with olive oil, sprinkle with dried herbs, salt, and pepper. Toss to coat evenly.

4. Roast in the preheated oven for 20-25 minutes, stirring halfway through, until vegetables are tender and lightly browned.

5. In a large bowl, combine cooked quinoa and roasted vegetables. Toss gently to combine.

6. If using, sprinkle with crumbled feta cheese and drizzle with balsamic glaze.

7. Serve warm or at room temperature as a satisfying salad option.

15. Lemon Garlic Shrimp with Broccoli and Brown Rice

Ingredients:

- 1 pound shrimp, peeled and deveined
- 2 tablespoons olive oil
- 4 cloves garlic, minced
- Zest and juice of 1 lemon
- Salt and pepper to taste
- 2 cups broccoli florets
- 2 cups cooked brown rice

Instructions:

1. In a large skillet, heat olive oil over medium heat. Add minced garlic and cook until fragrant, about 1 minute.

2. Add shrimp to the skillet, season with lemon zest, lemon juice, salt, and pepper. Cook until shrimp turn pink and opaque, about 2-3 minutes per side. Remove shrimp from skillet and set aside.

3. In the same skillet, add broccoli florets. Cook for 3-4 minutes until tender-crisp.

4. Return cooked shrimp to the skillet, toss with broccoli to combine.

5. Serve hot over cooked brown rice, garnished with additional lemon zest if desired.

16. Mixed Berry Smoothie Bowl

Ingredients:

- 1 cup mixed berries (such as strawberries, blueberries, raspberries)
- 1 ripe banana
- 1/2 cup Greek yogurt
- 1/4 cup almond milk (or any milk of choice)
- 1 tablespoon honey (optional)
- Toppings: sliced banana, granola, shredded coconut, chia seeds

Instructions:

1. In a blender, combine mixed berries, banana, Greek yogurt, almond milk, and honey. Blend until smooth and creamy.
2. Pour the smoothie into a bowl.
3. Top with sliced banana, granola, shredded coconut, and chia seeds.
4. Serve immediately with a spoon and enjoy this nutritious and delicious breakfast option.

17.Eggplant Parmesan

Ingredients:

- 1 large eggplant, sliced into rounds
- 2 eggs, beaten
- 1 cup breadcrumbs
- 1/2 cup grated Parmesan cheese
- 2 cups marinara sauce
- 1 cup shredded mozzarella cheese
- Fresh basil leaves for garnish
- Salt and pepper to taste

Instructions:

1. Preheat your oven to 375°F (190°C).
2. Dip eggplant slices into beaten eggs, then coat with breadcrumbs mixed with grated Parmesan cheese.
3. Place coated eggplant slices on a baking sheet lined with parchment paper.
4. Bake in the preheated oven for 20-25 minutes or until golden brown and crispy.
5. In a baking dish, spread a thin layer of marinara sauce. Place half of the baked eggplant slices on top.

6. Add another layer of marinara sauce and sprinkle with shredded mozzarella cheese.

7. Repeat the layers with the remaining ingredients.

8. Bake for an additional 15-20 minutes or until the cheese is melted and bubbly.

9. Garnish with fresh basil leaves before serving.

18. Tuna and White Bean Salad

Ingredients:

- 2 cans (5 ounces each) tuna, drained
- 1 can (15 ounces) white beans, drained and rinsed
- 1/4 cup red onion, finely chopped
- 1/4 cup celery, finely chopped
- 1/4 cup fresh parsley, chopped
- Juice of 1 lemon
- 2 tablespoons olive oil
- Salt and pepper to taste
- Optional: cherry tomatoes, sliced cucumber, mixed greens

Instructions:

1. In a large bowl, combine tuna, white beans, red onion, celery, and parsley.
2. In a small bowl, whisk together lemon juice, olive oil, salt, and pepper to make the dressing.
3. Pour the dressing over the tuna and white bean mixture. Toss gently to coat.
4. Serve as is or over a bed of mixed greens with sliced cherry tomatoes and cucumber for added freshness.

19.Vegetable Frittata

Ingredients:

- 8 large eggs
- 1/4 cup milk or cream
- 1 tablespoon olive oil
- 1 small onion, diced
- 1 bell pepper, diced
- 1 cup chopped spinach
- 1/2 cup cherry tomatoes, halved
- Salt and pepper to taste
- 1/4 cup shredded cheese (such as cheddar or feta)

Instructions:

1. Preheat your oven to 350°F (175°C).
2. In a bowl, whisk together eggs, milk, salt, and pepper until well combined.
3. In a large oven-safe skillet, heat olive oil over medium heat. Add diced onion and bell pepper, sauté until softened.
4. Add chopped spinach and cherry tomatoes to the skillet. Cook for another 2-3 minutes until spinach wilts.

5. Pour the egg mixture evenly over the vegetables in the skillet. Sprinkle shredded cheese on top.

6. Transfer the skillet to the preheated oven and bake for 15-20 minutes or until the frittata is set and the top is golden brown.

7. Slice into wedges and serve hot or at room temperature.

20. Mushroom and Spinach Stuffed Chicken Breast

Ingredients:

- 4 boneless, skinless chicken breasts
- Salt and pepper to taste
- 1 tablespoon olive oil
- 2 cups mushrooms, sliced
- 2 cups fresh spinach leaves
- 2 cloves garlic, minced
- 1/4 cup grated Parmesan cheese
- Toothpicks or kitchen twine

Instructions:

1. Preheat your oven to 375°F (190°C).

2. Season chicken breasts with salt and pepper. Slice a pocket into each chicken breast.

3. In a skillet, heat olive oil over medium heat. Add mushrooms and garlic, sauté until mushrooms are golden brown.

4. Add spinach to the skillet and cook until wilted. Remove from heat and stir in grated Parmesan cheese.

5. Stuff each chicken breast with the mushroom-spinach mixture. Secure with toothpicks or tie with kitchen twine to keep the stuffing in place.

6. Place stuffed chicken breasts on a baking sheet lined with parchment paper.

7. Bake in the preheated oven for 25-30 minutes or until chicken is cooked through and juices run clear.

8. Remove toothpicks or twine before serving.

21.Quinoa-Stuffed Bell Peppers

Ingredients:

- 4 large bell peppers, halved and seeds removed
- 1 cup quinoa, rinsed
- 2 cups vegetable broth
- 1 tablespoon olive oil
- 1 onion, diced
- 2 cloves garlic, minced
- 1 zucchini, diced
- 1 cup cherry tomatoes, halved
- 1/4 cup chopped fresh basil
- Salt and pepper to taste
- 1/2 cup shredded mozzarella cheese

Instructions:

1. Preheat your oven to 375°F (190°C).

2. In a medium saucepan, bring vegetable broth to a boil. Add quinoa, reduce heat to low, cover, and simmer for 15 minutes or until liquid is absorbed. Fluff with a fork and set aside.

3. In a skillet, heat olive oil over medium heat. Add diced onion and garlic, sauté until softened.

4. Add diced zucchini and cherry tomatoes to the skillet. Cook for 5-6 minutes until vegetables are tender.

5. Stir cooked quinoa and chopped fresh basil into the vegetable mixture. Season with salt and pepper to taste.

6. Arrange bell pepper halves in a baking dish. Spoon quinoa mixture into each pepper half.

7. Sprinkle shredded mozzarella cheese on top of each stuffed pepper.

8. Cover the baking dish with foil and bake in the preheated oven for 25-30 minutes or until peppers are tender and cheese is melted.

9. Serve hot as a satisfying and nutritious meal.

22. Turkey and Vegetable Skewers with Tzatziki Sauce

Ingredients:

- 1 pound turkey breast, cut into chunks
- 1 red bell pepper, cut into chunks
- 1 yellow bell pepper, cut into chunks
- 1 red onion, cut into chunks
- 1 zucchini, sliced
- Wooden skewers, soaked in water for 30 minutes
- Salt and pepper to taste
- Olive oil for brushing

For the Tzatziki Sauce:

- 1 cup Greek yogurt
- 1/2 cucumber, grated and squeezed to remove excess moisture
- 1 clove garlic, minced
- 1 tablespoon lemon juice
- 1 tablespoon chopped fresh dill
- Salt and pepper to taste

Instructions:

1. Preheat your grill or grill pan over medium-high heat.

2. Thread turkey chunks, bell pepper chunks, onion chunks, and zucchini slices alternately onto the soaked wooden skewers.

3. Brush the skewers with olive oil and season with salt and pepper.

4. Grill the skewers for 8-10 minutes, turning occasionally, until turkey is cooked through and vegetables are tender and lightly charred.

5. While the skewers are grilling, prepare the tzatziki sauce by combining Greek yogurt, grated cucumber, minced garlic, lemon juice, chopped dill, salt, and pepper in a bowl. Mix well.

6. Serve the grilled turkey and vegetable skewers hot with tzatziki sauce on the side for dipping.

23.Creamy Tomato Basil Soup

Ingredients:

- 2 tablespoons olive oil

- 1 onion, chopped

- 2 cloves garlic, minced

- 2 cans (14 ounces each) diced tomatoes

- 1 can (14 ounces) tomato sauce

- 2 cups vegetable broth

- 1/2 cup heavy cream or coconut cream

- 1/4 cup chopped fresh basil leaves

- Salt and pepper to taste

- Optional: grated Parmesan cheese and additional fresh basil for garnish

Instructions:

1. In a large pot, heat olive oil over medium heat. Add chopped onion and minced garlic, sauté until softened.

2. Add diced tomatoes, tomato sauce, and vegetable broth to the pot. Bring to a simmer and cook for 15-20 minutes.

3. Using an immersion blender or transferring the mixture to a blender, blend until smooth.

4. Return the soup to the pot over low heat. Stir in heavy cream and chopped fresh basil. Season with salt and pepper to taste.

5. Let the soup simmer for an additional 5 minutes.

6. Serve hot, garnished with grated Parmesan cheese and additional fresh basil if desired.

24. Turkey and Vegetable Stir-Fry with Brown Rice

Ingredients:

- 1 tablespoon vegetable oil

- 1 pound turkey breast, sliced into strips

- 2 cups mixed vegetables (such as bell peppers, broccoli, carrots, snap peas)

- 3 cloves garlic, minced

- 1 tablespoon grated ginger

- 1/4 cup low-sodium soy sauce

- 2 tablespoons hoisin sauce

- 1 tablespoon honey

- 2 cups cooked brown rice

Instructions:

1. Heat vegetable oil in a large skillet or wok over high heat.

2. Add turkey strips and cook until browned and cooked through, about 5-6 minutes. Remove from skillet and set aside.

3. In the same skillet, add mixed vegetables, minced garlic, and grated ginger. Stir-fry for 3-4 minutes until vegetables are tender-crisp.

4. Return cooked turkey to the skillet. Add soy sauce, hoisin sauce, and honey. Stir to combine and heat through.

5. Serve hot over cooked brown rice.

25. Blueberry Banana Oat Muffins

Ingredients:

- 1 cup rolled oats
- 1 cup whole wheat flour
- 1 teaspoon baking powder
- 1/2 teaspoon baking soda
- 1/4 teaspoon salt
- 2 ripe bananas, mashed
- 1/4 cup honey or maple syrup
- 1/4 cup milk or non-dairy milk
- 1/4 cup Greek yogurt
- 1 egg
- 1 teaspoon vanilla extract
- 1 cup fresh or frozen blueberries

Instructions:

1. Preheat your oven to 350°F (175°C). Line a muffin tin with paper liners or grease with cooking spray.

2. In a large bowl, mix together rolled oats, whole wheat flour, baking powder, baking soda, and salt.

3. In another bowl, whisk together mashed bananas, honey or maple syrup, milk, Greek yogurt, egg, and vanilla extract until well combined.

4. Pour the wet ingredients into the dry ingredients and stir until just combined. Gently fold in the blueberries.

5. Divide the batter evenly among the prepared muffin cups.

6. Bake in the preheated oven for 18-20 minutes or until a toothpick inserted into the center comes out clean.

7. Allow the muffins to cool in the pan for 5 minutes before transferring to a wire rack to cool completely.

26.Salmon and Vegetable Foil Packets

Ingredients:

- 4 salmon fillets
- 2 cups mixed vegetables (such as bell peppers, zucchini, cherry tomatoes)
- 4 tablespoons olive oil
- 4 cloves garlic, minced
- 2 tablespoons lemon juice
- Salt and pepper to taste
- Fresh herbs for garnish (such as parsley or dill)

Instructions:

1. Preheat your oven to 375°F (190°C).
2. Cut four pieces of aluminum foil, each large enough to wrap a salmon fillet and vegetables.
3. Place a salmon fillet on each piece of foil. Arrange mixed vegetables around the salmon.
4. In a small bowl, whisk together olive oil, minced garlic, lemon juice, salt, and pepper.
5. Drizzle the olive oil mixture over the salmon and vegetables.
6. Fold the foil over the salmon and vegetables, crimping the edges to seal tightly.

7. Place the foil packets on a baking sheet and bake in the preheated oven for 15-20 minutes, or until the salmon is cooked through and the vegetables are tender.

8. Carefully open the foil packets, garnish with fresh herbs, and serve hot.

27.Black Bean and Corn Salad

Ingredients:

- 2 cans (15 ounces each) black beans, drained and rinsed
- 1 cup frozen corn, thawed
- 1 red bell pepper, diced
- 1/2 red onion, finely chopped
- 1/4 cup chopped fresh cilantro
- Juice of 2 limes
- 2 tablespoons olive oil
- 1 teaspoon ground cumin
- Salt and pepper to taste
- Optional: diced avocado for garnish

Instructions:

1. In a large bowl, combine black beans, corn, diced red bell pepper, chopped red onion, and fresh cilantro.

2. In a small bowl, whisk together lime juice, olive oil, ground cumin, salt, and pepper.

3. Pour the dressing over the black bean mixture and toss to combine.

4. Taste and adjust seasoning if needed.

5. If desired, garnish with diced avocado before serving.

6. Serve chilled as a refreshing salad or as a side dish with grilled chicken or fish.

28.Sweet Potato and Chickpea Buddha Bowl

Ingredients:

- 2 large sweet potatoes, peeled and cubed

- 1 can (15 ounces) chickpeas, drained and rinsed

- 2 tablespoons olive oil

- 1 teaspoon ground cumin

- 1 teaspoon smoked paprika

- Salt and pepper to taste

- 4 cups cooked quinoa or brown rice

- 2 cups baby spinach or mixed greens

- 1 avocado, sliced

- Tahini dressing or your favorite dressing for drizzling

Instructions:

1. Preheat your oven to 400°F (200°C).

2. Place cubed sweet potatoes and chickpeas on a baking sheet lined with parchment paper.

3. Drizzle with olive oil and sprinkle with ground cumin, smoked paprika, salt, and pepper. Toss to coat evenly.

4. Roast in the preheated oven for 25-30 minutes, stirring halfway through, until sweet potatoes are tender and chickpeas are crispy.

5. Divide cooked quinoa or brown rice among serving bowls. Top with roasted sweet potatoes and chickpeas.

6. Add baby spinach or mixed greens to each bowl.

7. Garnish with sliced avocado.

8. Drizzle with tahini dressing or your favorite dressing before serving.

29.Vegetable and Lentil Curry

Ingredients:

- 1 tablespoon olive oil
- 1 onion, diced
- 2 cloves garlic, minced
- 1 tablespoon grated ginger
- 2 carrots, diced
- 2 potatoes, peeled and diced
- 1 cup dried red lentils, rinsed
- 1 can (14 ounces) diced tomatoes
- 1 can (14 ounces) coconut milk
- 2 cups vegetable broth
- 2 tablespoons curry powder
- 1 teaspoon ground turmeric
- Salt and pepper to taste
- Fresh cilantro for garnish

Instructions:

1. In a large pot, heat olive oil over medium heat. Add diced onion, minced garlic, and grated ginger. Sauté until fragrant and onions are translucent.

2. Add diced carrots and potatoes to the pot. Cook for 5 minutes, stirring occasionally.

3. Stir in rinsed red lentils, diced tomatoes, coconut milk, vegetable broth, curry powder, ground turmeric, salt, and pepper.

4. Bring the mixture to a boil, then reduce heat to low and let simmer for 20-25 minutes, or until lentils and vegetables are tender and the curry has thickened.

5. Taste and adjust seasoning if necessary.

6. Serve hot, garnished with fresh cilantro. This curry pairs well with rice or naan bread.

30.Chicken and Quinoa Soup

Ingredients:

- 1 tablespoon olive oil
- 1 onion, diced
- 2 carrots, diced
- 2 celery stalks, diced
- 2 cloves garlic, minced
- 1 teaspoon dried thyme
- 1 teaspoon dried oregano
- 1/2 teaspoon paprika
- 1 cup quinoa, rinsed
- 6 cups chicken broth
- 2 cups cooked shredded chicken
- Salt and pepper to taste
- Fresh parsley for garnish

Instructions:

1. In a large pot, heat olive oil over medium heat. Add diced onion, carrots, and celery. Sauté until vegetables are softened, about 5 minutes.

2. Add minced garlic, dried thyme, dried oregano, and paprika. Cook for an additional 1-2 minutes until fragrant.

3. Stir in rinsed quinoa and chicken broth. Bring to a boil, then reduce heat to low and let simmer for 15-20 minutes, or until quinoa is cooked and vegetables are tender.

4. Add shredded chicken to the pot and simmer for another 5 minutes to heat through.

5. Season with salt and pepper to taste.

6. Serve hot, garnished with fresh parsley.

31. Apple Cinnamon Baked Oatmeal

Ingredients:

- 2 cups old-fashioned rolled oats
- 1 teaspoon baking powder
- 1 teaspoon ground cinnamon
- 1/4 teaspoon salt
- 1 1/2 cups milk or non-dairy milk
- 1/4 cup maple syrup
- 2 tablespoons melted butter or coconut oil
- 1 large egg
- 1 teaspoon vanilla extract
- 1 apple, peeled, cored, and diced
- Optional toppings: chopped nuts, raisins, additional maple syrup

Instructions:

1. Preheat your oven to 350°F (175°C). Grease a baking dish with butter or cooking spray.

2. In a large bowl, mix together rolled oats, baking powder, ground cinnamon, and salt.

3. In another bowl, whisk together milk, maple syrup, melted butter or coconut oil, egg, and vanilla extract until well combined.

4. Pour the wet ingredients into the dry ingredients and stir until fully incorporated.

5. Gently fold in diced apple.

6. Pour the mixture into the prepared baking dish.

7. Bake in the preheated oven for 30-35 minutes, or until the top is golden brown and the oatmeal is set.

8. Serve warm, optionally topped with chopped nuts, raisins, and additional maple syrup.

32.Turkey and Vegetable Meatloaf

Ingredients:

- 1 pound ground turkey

- 1 onion, finely chopped

- 2 cloves garlic, minced

- 1 carrot, grated

- 1 zucchini, grated

- 1/2 cup rolled oats

- 1/4 cup ketchup

- 2 tablespoons Worcestershire sauce

- 1 tablespoon Dijon mustard

- 1 teaspoon dried thyme

- Salt and pepper to taste

- Optional: barbecue sauce for topping

Instructions:

1. Preheat your oven to 375°F (190°C). Grease a loaf pan with cooking spray.

2. In a large bowl, combine ground turkey, chopped onion, minced garlic, grated carrot, grated zucchini, rolled oats, ketchup, Worcestershire sauce, Dijon mustard, dried thyme, salt, and pepper.

3. Mix until all ingredients are well combined.

4. Transfer the mixture to the prepared loaf pan, pressing it down evenly.

5. If desired, spread a layer of barbecue sauce over the top of the meatloaf.

6. Bake in the preheated oven for 45-50 minutes, or until the meatloaf is cooked through and the top is golden brown.

7. Let the meatloaf cool for a few minutes before slicing and serving.

33.Greek Yogurt Chicken Salad

Ingredients:

- 2 cups cooked shredded chicken
- 1/2 cup Greek yogurt
- 1/4 cup diced celery
- 1/4 cup diced red onion
- 1/4 cup sliced almonds
- 1/4 cup dried cranberries
- 1 tablespoon lemon juice
- 1 teaspoon Dijon mustard
- Salt and pepper to taste
- Lettuce leaves or whole grain bread for serving

Instructions:

1. In a large bowl, combine shredded chicken, Greek yogurt, diced celery, diced red onion, sliced almonds, dried cranberries, lemon juice, Dijon mustard, salt, and pepper.

2. Mix until all ingredients are well coated with the yogurt mixture.

3. Serve the chicken salad on lettuce leaves for a low-carb option or on whole grain bread for a sandwich.

4. Enjoy immediately or refrigerate for later use.

34. Banana Chocolate Chip Muffins

Ingredients:

- 2 cups all-purpose flour
- 1 teaspoon baking powder
- 1/2 teaspoon baking soda
- 1/4 teaspoon salt
- 1/2 cup unsalted butter, melted
- 3/4 cup granulated sugar
- 2 ripe bananas, mashed
- 1/2 cup Greek yogurt
- 1 large egg
- 1 teaspoon vanilla extract
- 1/2 cup chocolate chips

Instructions:

1. Preheat your oven to 350°F (175°C). Line a muffin tin with paper liners or grease with cooking spray.

2. In a large bowl, whisk together all-purpose flour, baking powder, baking soda, and salt.

3. In another bowl, mix melted butter and granulated sugar until well combined.

4. Add mashed bananas, Greek yogurt, egg, and vanilla extract to the butter-sugar mixture. Mix until smooth.

5. Gradually add the dry ingredients to the wet ingredients, stirring until just combined.

6. Gently fold in chocolate chips.

7. Divide the batter evenly among the prepared muffin cups.

8. Bake in the preheated oven for 18-20 minutes, or until a toothpick inserted into the center of a muffin comes out clean.

9. Allow the muffins to cool in the pan for 5 minutes before transferring to a wire rack to cool completely.

35.Vegetable and Lentil Soup

Ingredients:

- 1 tablespoon olive oil

- 1 onion, diced

- 2 carrots, diced

- 2 celery stalks, diced

- 2 cloves garlic, minced

- 1 teaspoon dried thyme

- 1 teaspoon dried rosemary

- 1 cup dried green or brown lentils, rinsed

- 4 cups vegetable broth

- 2 cups water

- 1 can (14 ounces) diced tomatoes

- Salt and pepper to taste

- Fresh parsley for garnish

Instructions:

1. Heat olive oil in a large pot over medium heat. Add diced onion, carrots, and celery. Cook until vegetables are softened, about 5 minutes.

2. Add minced garlic, dried thyme, and dried rosemary. Cook for another minute until fragrant.

3. Stir in rinsed lentils, vegetable broth, water, and diced tomatoes with their juices. Bring to a boil.

4. Reduce heat to low, cover, and simmer for 20-25 minutes or until lentils are tender.

5. Season with salt and pepper to taste.

6. Serve hot, garnished with fresh parsley.

36. Caprese Quinoa Salad

Ingredients:

- 1 cup quinoa, rinsed

- 2 cups water

- 1 pint cherry tomatoes, halved

- 8 ounces fresh mozzarella cheese, diced

- 1/4 cup chopped fresh basil

- 2 tablespoons extra virgin olive oil

- 1 tablespoon balsamic vinegar

- Salt and pepper to taste

Instructions:

1. In a medium saucepan, combine quinoa and water. Bring to a boil, then reduce heat to low, cover, and simmer for 15-20 minutes or until quinoa is cooked and water is absorbed. Fluff with a fork and let cool.

2. In a large bowl, combine cooked quinoa, halved cherry tomatoes, diced fresh mozzarella, and chopped fresh basil.

3. Drizzle with extra virgin olive oil and balsamic vinegar. Toss to combine.

4. Season with salt and pepper to taste.

5. Serve chilled or at room temperature as a refreshing salad option.

37.Honey Mustard Glazed Salmon

Ingredients:

- 4 salmon fillets

- Salt and pepper to taste

- 1/4 cup honey

- 2 tablespoons Dijon mustard

- 1 tablespoon soy sauce

- 1 tablespoon olive oil

- 2 cloves garlic, minced

- 1 teaspoon grated ginger

- Sesame seeds for garnish

- Sliced green onions for garnish

Instructions:

1. Preheat your oven to 400°F (200°C). Line a baking sheet with parchment paper.

2. Season salmon fillets with salt and pepper. Place them on the prepared baking sheet.

3. In a small bowl, whisk together honey, Dijon mustard, soy sauce, olive oil, minced garlic, and grated ginger.

4. Brush the honey mustard glaze over the salmon fillets, coating them evenly.

5. Bake in the preheated oven for 12-15 minutes, or until the salmon is cooked through and flakes easily with a fork.

6. Sprinkle with sesame seeds and sliced green onions before serving.

38. Quinoa and Black Bean Stuffed Bell Peppers

Ingredients:

- 4 large bell peppers, halved and seeds removed
- 1 cup quinoa, rinsed
- 2 cups vegetable broth
- 1 tablespoon olive oil
- 1 onion, diced
- 2 cloves garlic, minced
- 1 can (15 ounces) black beans, drained and rinsed
- 1 cup corn kernels (fresh, frozen, or canned)

- 1 teaspoon ground cumin

- 1 teaspoon chili powder

- Salt and pepper to taste

- Optional toppings: shredded cheese, chopped cilantro, avocado slices

Instructions:

1. Preheat your oven to 375°F (190°C).

2. In a medium saucepan, bring vegetable broth to a boil. Add quinoa, reduce heat to low, cover, and simmer for 15 minutes or until liquid is absorbed. Fluff with a fork and set aside.

3. Heat olive oil in a large skillet over medium heat. Add diced onion and minced garlic, sauté until softened.

4. Add cooked quinoa, black beans, corn kernels, ground cumin, chili powder, salt, and pepper to the skillet. Stir to combine and cook for 5 minutes.

5. Arrange bell pepper halves in a baking dish. Spoon quinoa and black bean mixture into each pepper half.

6. Cover the baking dish with foil and bake in the preheated oven for 25-30 minutes or until peppers are tender.

7. If desired, top stuffed peppers with shredded cheese, chopped cilantro, and avocado slices before serving.

39.Mango and Avocado Salad

Ingredients:

- 2 ripe mangoes, peeled, pitted, and diced

- 2 ripe avocados, peeled, pitted, and diced

- 1/4 cup red onion, finely chopped

- 1/4 cup chopped fresh cilantro

- Juice of 1 lime

- 1 tablespoon extra virgin olive oil

- Salt and pepper to taste

- Optional: diced jalapeño for heat, crumbled feta cheese for tanginess

Instructions:

1. In a large bowl, combine diced mangoes, diced avocados, finely chopped red onion, and chopped fresh cilantro.

2. Drizzle lime juice and extra virgin olive oil over the salad. Season with salt and pepper to taste.

3. Toss gently to combine all ingredients.

4. If desired, add diced jalapeño for extra heat or crumbled feta cheese for tanginess.

5. Serve immediately as a refreshing side dish or as a topping for grilled chicken or fish.

40. Turkey and Vegetable Stir-Fry with Rice Noodles

Ingredients:

- 8 ounces rice noodles
- 1 tablespoon vegetable oil
- 1 pound ground turkey
- 2 cloves garlic, minced
- 1 tablespoon grated ginger
- 1 bell pepper, sliced
- 1 cup snap peas
- 1 carrot, julienned
- 1/4 cup low-sodium soy sauce
- 2 tablespoons hoisin sauce
- 1 tablespoon rice vinegar

- 1 teaspoon sesame oil

- Optional toppings: sliced green onions, sesame seeds

Instructions:

1. Cook rice noodles according to package instructions. Drain and set aside.

2. Heat vegetable oil in a large skillet or wok over medium-high heat. Add ground turkey and cook until browned and cooked through.

3. Add minced garlic and grated ginger to the skillet, stir-fry for 1 minute until fragrant.

4. Add sliced bell pepper, snap peas, and julienned carrot to the skillet. Stir-fry for 3-4 minutes until vegetables are tender-crisp.

5. In a small bowl, whisk together low-sodium soy sauce, hoisin sauce, rice vinegar, and sesame oil. Pour the sauce over the turkey and vegetable mixture in the skillet.

6. Add cooked rice noodles to the skillet and toss to coat everything evenly with the sauce.

7. Cook for an additional 2-3 minutes until heated through.

8. Serve hot, garnished with sliced green onions and sesame seeds if desired.

41.Spinach and Feta Stuffed Chicken Breast

Ingredients:

- 4 boneless, skinless chicken breasts
- Salt and pepper to taste
- 2 cups fresh spinach leaves
- 1/2 cup crumbled feta cheese
- 1 tablespoon olive oil
- 2 cloves garlic, minced
- 1/2 teaspoon dried oregano
- 1/2 teaspoon dried basil
- Toothpicks or kitchen twine

Instructions:

1. Preheat your oven to 375°F (190°C).
2. Use a sharp knife to cut a pocket into the side of each chicken breast, being careful not to cut all the way through.
3. Season the chicken breasts with salt and pepper, both inside and out.
4. In a skillet, heat olive oil over medium heat. Add minced garlic and sauté until fragrant, about 1 minute.

5. Add fresh spinach leaves to the skillet and cook until wilted.

6. Remove the skillet from heat and stir in crumbled feta cheese, dried oregano, and dried basil.

7. Stuff each chicken breast with the spinach and feta mixture, then secure the opening with toothpicks or tie with kitchen twine.

8. Place the stuffed chicken breasts in a baking dish and bake in the preheated oven for 25-30 minutes, or until chicken is cooked through and no longer pink in the center.

9. Remove toothpicks or twine before serving.

42. Quinoa and Vegetable Stuffed Portobello Mushrooms

Ingredients:

- 4 large portobello mushrooms, stems removed
- 1 cup cooked quinoa
- 1 cup diced bell peppers (any color)
- 1/2 cup diced zucchini
- 1/2 cup diced red onion
- 2 cloves garlic, minced

- 1 tablespoon olive oil

- 1/4 cup grated Parmesan cheese

- Salt and pepper to taste

- Fresh parsley for garnish

Instructions:

1. Preheat your oven to 375°F (190°C).

2. Place portobello mushrooms on a baking sheet lined with parchment paper, gill-side up.

3. In a skillet, heat olive oil over medium heat. Add diced bell peppers, diced zucchini, diced red onion, and minced garlic. Sauté until vegetables are tender.

4. Stir in cooked quinoa and grated Parmesan cheese. Season with salt and pepper to taste.

5. Divide the quinoa and vegetable mixture among the portobello mushrooms, filling each mushroom cap generously.

6. Bake in the preheated oven for 20-25 minutes, or until mushrooms are tender and filling is heated through.

7. Garnish with fresh parsley before serving.

43.Banana Berry Smoothie

Ingredients:

- 2 ripe bananas, peeled and frozen

- 1 cup mixed berries (such as strawberries, blueberries, raspberries)

- 1 cup spinach leaves

- 1 cup Greek yogurt

- 1 tablespoon honey or maple syrup (optional)

- 1 cup almond milk or any milk of choice

Instructions:

1. Place frozen bananas, mixed berries, spinach leaves, Greek yogurt, honey or maple syrup (if using), and almond milk in a blender.

2. Blend until smooth and creamy, adding more milk if needed to reach your desired consistency.

3. Taste and adjust sweetness if necessary by adding more honey or maple syrup.

4. Pour into glasses and serve immediately for a refreshing and nutritious smoothie option.

44. Broccoli and Cheddar Stuffed Baked Potatoes

Ingredients:

- 4 large russet potatoes

- 2 cups broccoli florets, steamed

- 1 cup shredded cheddar cheese

- 1/2 cup sour cream

- 2 tablespoons butter

- Salt and pepper to taste

- Optional toppings: chopped chives, crispy bacon bits

Instructions:

1. Preheat your oven to 400°F (200°C).

2. Scrub the potatoes clean and pat them dry. Pierce each potato several times with a fork.

3. Place the potatoes directly on the oven rack and bake for 45-60 minutes, or until tender when pierced with a fork.

4. While the potatoes are baking, steam the broccoli florets until tender.

5. Once the potatoes are baked, carefully slice each one open lengthwise and fluff the insides with a fork.

6. Divide steamed broccoli among the potatoes, then top with shredded cheddar cheese, sour cream, and butter.

7. Season with salt and pepper to taste.

8. If desired, sprinkle chopped chives and crispy bacon bits over the top.

9. Serve hot as a comforting and satisfying meal.

45. Mediterranean Chickpea Salad

Ingredients:

- 2 cans (15 ounces each) chickpeas, drained and rinsed

- 1 cup cherry tomatoes, halved

- 1 cucumber, diced

- 1/2 red onion, thinly sliced

- 1/4 cup chopped fresh parsley

- 1/4 cup chopped fresh mint

- 1/4 cup crumbled feta cheese

- Juice of 1 lemon

- 2 tablespoons extra virgin olive oil

- Salt and pepper to taste

Instructions:

1. In a large bowl, combine chickpeas, cherry tomatoes, diced cucumber, thinly sliced red onion, chopped fresh parsley, and chopped fresh mint.

2. Add crumbled feta cheese to the bowl.

3. Drizzle lemon juice and extra virgin olive oil over the salad. Season with salt and pepper to taste.

4. Toss gently to combine all ingredients.

5. Serve chilled or at room temperature as a refreshing and flavorful salad option.

46.Turkey and Vegetable Lettuce Wraps

Ingredients:

- 1 tablespoon olive oil

- 1 pound ground turkey

- 1 bell pepper, diced

- 1 carrot, grated

- 2 cloves garlic, minced

- 2 green onions, thinly sliced

- 2 tablespoons hoisin sauce

- 1 tablespoon soy sauce
- 1 teaspoon sesame oil
- 1/4 cup chopped peanuts (optional)
- Butter lettuce leaves for wrapping

Instructions:

1. Heat olive oil in a large skillet over medium heat. Add ground turkey and cook until browned.

2. Add diced bell pepper, grated carrot, minced garlic, and sliced green onions to the skillet. Cook for 3-4 minutes until vegetables are tender.

3. Stir in hoisin sauce, soy sauce, and sesame oil. Cook for an additional 2 minutes.

4. If using chopped peanuts, sprinkle them over the turkey and vegetable mixture and toss to combine.

5. Spoon the turkey and vegetable mixture onto butter lettuce leaves.

6. Serve the lettuce wraps immediately, allowing everyone to assemble their own wraps.

47.Sautéed Shrimp with Garlic and Lemon

Ingredients:

- 1 pound large shrimp, peeled and deveined
- Salt and pepper to taste
- 2 tablespoons olive oil
- 4 cloves garlic, minced
- Zest and juice of 1 lemon
- 2 tablespoons chopped fresh parsley
- Lemon wedges for serving

Instructions:

1. Pat the shrimp dry with paper towels and season with salt and pepper.
2. Heat olive oil in a large skillet over medium-high heat.
3. Add minced garlic to the skillet and sauté for 1 minute until fragrant.
4. Add the seasoned shrimp to the skillet in a single layer and cook for 2-3 minutes per side until pink and cooked through.
5. Stir in lemon zest and juice, and chopped fresh parsley.
6. Serve hot, garnished with lemon wedges.

48.Quinoa and Vegetable Stir-Fry

Ingredients:

- 1 cup quinoa, rinsed
- 2 cups water or vegetable broth
- 2 tablespoons soy sauce
- 1 tablespoon hoisin sauce
- 1 tablespoon rice vinegar
- 1 tablespoon sesame oil
- 1 tablespoon vegetable oil
- 2 cloves garlic, minced
- 1 tablespoon grated ginger
- 1 bell pepper, thinly sliced
- 1 cup broccoli florets
- 1 cup sliced mushrooms
- 1 cup snap peas
- Salt and pepper to taste
- Optional toppings: sliced green onions, sesame seeds

Instructions:

1. In a medium saucepan, combine quinoa and water or vegetable broth. Bring to a boil, then reduce

heat to low, cover, and simmer for 15-20 minutes until quinoa is cooked and liquid is absorbed.

2. In a small bowl, whisk together soy sauce, hoisin sauce, rice vinegar, and sesame oil. Set aside.

3. Heat vegetable oil in a large skillet or wok over medium-high heat.

4. Add minced garlic and grated ginger to the skillet and sauté for 1 minute until fragrant.

5. Add sliced bell pepper, broccoli florets, sliced mushrooms, and snap peas to the skillet. Stir-fry for 4-5 minutes until vegetables are tender-crisp.

6. Stir in cooked quinoa and the prepared sauce. Cook for an additional 2-3 minutes to heat through.

7. Season with salt and pepper to taste.

8. Serve hot, garnished with sliced green onions and sesame seeds if desired.

49.Oven-Roasted Brussels Sprouts

Ingredients:

- 1 pound Brussels sprouts, trimmed and halved

- 2 tablespoons olive oil

- Salt and pepper to taste

- Optional toppings: grated Parmesan cheese, balsamic glaze

Instructions:

1. Preheat your oven to 400°F (200°C). Line a baking sheet with parchment paper.

2. Place halved Brussels sprouts on the prepared baking sheet.

3. Drizzle olive oil over the Brussels sprouts and toss to coat evenly.

4. Season with salt and pepper to taste.

5. Roast in the preheated oven for 20-25 minutes, stirring halfway through, until Brussels sprouts are golden brown and tender.

6. If desired, sprinkle grated Parmesan cheese over the roasted Brussels sprouts before serving.

7. Drizzle with balsamic glaze for extra flavor.

50.Vegetarian Lentil Soup

Ingredients:

- 1 cup dried lentils, rinsed
- 4 cups vegetable broth
- 1 onion, diced
- 2 carrots, diced
- 2 celery stalks, diced
- 2 cloves garlic, minced
- 1 can (14 ounces) diced tomatoes
- 1 teaspoon dried thyme
- 1 teaspoon dried oregano
- Salt and pepper to taste
- 2 tablespoons olive oil
- Fresh parsley for garnish

Instructions:

1. In a large pot, heat olive oil over medium heat. Add diced onion, carrots, and celery. Sauté until vegetables are softened, about 5 minutes.

2. Add minced garlic to the pot and cook for another minute until fragrant.

3. Stir in rinsed lentils, vegetable broth, diced tomatoes with their juices, dried thyme, and dried oregano.

4. Bring the soup to a boil, then reduce heat to low and let it simmer for about 25-30 minutes, or until lentils are tender.

5. Season with salt and pepper to taste.

6. Serve hot, garnished with fresh parsley.

51. Grilled Lemon Herb Chicken

Ingredients:

- 4 boneless, skinless chicken breasts
- Zest and juice of 2 lemons
- 2 cloves garlic, minced
- 2 tablespoons chopped fresh parsley
- 1 tablespoon chopped fresh thyme
- 1 tablespoon olive oil
- Salt and pepper to taste

Instructions:

1. In a bowl, combine lemon zest, lemon juice, minced garlic, chopped fresh parsley, chopped fresh thyme, olive oil, salt, and pepper.

2. Place the chicken breasts in a shallow dish and pour the marinade over them, turning to coat evenly.

3. Cover the dish and refrigerate for at least 30 minutes, or up to 4 hours.

4. Preheat grill to medium-high heat. Remove chicken from marinade and discard any excess marinade.

5. Grill chicken breasts for 6-8 minutes per side, or until cooked through and juices run clear.

6. Remove from grill and let rest for a few minutes before serving.

52.Berry and Spinach Smoothie Bowl

Ingredients:

- 1 ripe banana, peeled and frozen
- 1 cup mixed berries (such as strawberries, blueberries, raspberries)
- 1 cup fresh spinach leaves
- 1/2 cup Greek yogurt
- 1/4 cup almond milk or any milk of choice
- Toppings: sliced strawberries, blueberries, granola, shredded coconut, chia seeds

Instructions:

1. In a blender, combine frozen banana, mixed berries, fresh spinach leaves, Greek yogurt, and almond milk.
2. Blend until smooth and creamy, adding more milk if needed to reach desired consistency.
3. Pour the smoothie into a bowl.
4. Top with sliced strawberries, blueberries, granola, shredded coconut, and chia seeds.
5. Serve immediately and enjoy with a spoon.

53. Sweet Potato and Black Bean Tacos

Ingredients:

- 2 large sweet potatoes, peeled and diced
- 1 tablespoon olive oil
- 1 teaspoon ground cumin
- 1 teaspoon chili powder
- 1/2 teaspoon smoked paprika
- Salt and pepper to taste
- 1 can (15 ounces) black beans, drained and rinsed
- 8 small corn tortillas
- Toppings: shredded lettuce, diced tomatoes, sliced avocado, chopped cilantro, lime wedges

Instructions:

1. Preheat your oven to 400°F (200°C).
2. Place diced sweet potatoes on a baking sheet lined with parchment paper.
3. Drizzle olive oil over the sweet potatoes and sprinkle with ground cumin, chili powder, smoked paprika, salt, and pepper. Toss to coat evenly.
4. Roast sweet potatoes in the preheated oven for 20-25 minutes, or until tender and lightly browned.

5. In a small saucepan, heat black beans over medium heat until warmed through.

6. Warm corn tortillas in a skillet or directly over a gas flame until heated through and slightly charred.

7. Assemble tacos by filling each tortilla with roasted sweet potatoes and black beans.

8. Top with shredded lettuce, diced tomatoes, sliced avocado, chopped cilantro, and a squeeze of lime juice.

9. Serve hot and enjoy your flavorful vegetarian tacos!

54. Honey Garlic Glazed Salmon

Ingredients:

- 4 salmon fillets

- Salt and pepper to taste

- 2 tablespoons honey

- 2 tablespoons soy sauce

- 2 cloves garlic, minced

- 1 tablespoon rice vinegar

- 1 tablespoon olive oil

- Optional garnish: sliced green onions, sesame seeds

Instructions:

1. Season salmon fillets with salt and pepper on both sides.

2. In a small bowl, whisk together honey, soy sauce, minced garlic, and rice vinegar to make the glaze.

3. Heat olive oil in a skillet over medium-high heat.

4. Place salmon fillets in the skillet, skin-side down, and cook for 3-4 minutes until golden brown and crispy.

5. Flip the salmon fillets and pour the honey garlic glaze over them.

6. Continue cooking for another 3-4 minutes, basting the salmon with the glaze, until salmon is cooked through and glazed.

7. Garnish with sliced green onions and sesame seeds if desired.

8. Serve hot, accompanied by your favorite side dishes.

55.Mango Avocado Salsa

Ingredients:

- 1 ripe mango, peeled and diced
- 1 ripe avocado, peeled, pitted, and diced
- 1/4 cup diced red onion
- 1/4 cup chopped fresh cilantro
- Juice of 1 lime
- Salt and pepper to taste

Instructions:

1. In a bowl, combine diced mango, diced avocado, diced red onion, chopped cilantro, and lime juice.
2. Gently toss to combine all ingredients.
3. Season with salt and pepper to taste.
4. Serve immediately as a topping for grilled chicken, fish, tacos, or as a dip with tortilla chips.

56.Vegetable and Tofu Stir-Fry

Ingredients:

- 14 ounces (400g) firm tofu, drained and pressed
- 2 tablespoons soy sauce
- 1 tablespoon rice vinegar
- 1 tablespoon sesame oil
- 1 tablespoon cornstarch
- 2 tablespoons vegetable oil
- 2 cloves garlic, minced
- 1 tablespoon grated ginger
- 1 bell pepper, sliced
- 1 cup broccoli florets
- 1 carrot, julienned
- 1 cup snap peas
- Salt and pepper to taste
- Cooked rice or noodles for serving

Instructions:

1. Cut the pressed tofu into cubes and place them in a bowl.

2. In a separate bowl, whisk together soy sauce, rice vinegar, sesame oil, and cornstarch to make the sauce.

3. Pour the sauce over the tofu cubes and toss to coat evenly.

4. Heat vegetable oil in a large skillet or wok over medium-high heat.

5. Add minced garlic and grated ginger to the skillet and sauté for 1 minute until fragrant.

6. Add sliced bell pepper, broccoli florets, julienned carrot, and snap peas to the skillet. Stir-fry for 4-5 minutes until vegetables are tender-crisp.

7. Push the vegetables to one side of the skillet and add the marinated tofu cubes to the other side.

8. Cook the tofu for 2-3 minutes on each side until golden brown and crispy.

9. Combine the tofu with the vegetables in the skillet and toss to mix.

10. Season with salt and pepper to taste.

11. Serve hot over cooked rice or noodles.

57.Roasted Vegetable Quinoa Bowl

Ingredients:

- 1 cup quinoa, rinsed

- 2 cups vegetable broth or water

- 2 cups chopped mixed vegetables (such as bell peppers, zucchini, eggplant, cherry tomatoes)

- 2 tablespoons olive oil

- 2 cloves garlic, minced

- 1 teaspoon dried thyme

- 1 teaspoon dried oregano

- Salt and pepper to taste

- Optional toppings: crumbled feta cheese, chopped fresh herbs, balsamic glaze

Instructions:

1. Preheat your oven to 400°F (200°C).

2. In a saucepan, combine quinoa and vegetable broth or water. Bring to a boil, then reduce heat to low, cover, and simmer for 15-20 minutes until quinoa is cooked and liquid is absorbed.

3. Spread chopped mixed vegetables on a baking sheet lined with parchment paper.

4. Drizzle olive oil over the vegetables and sprinkle with minced garlic, dried thyme, dried oregano, salt, and pepper. Toss to coat evenly.

5. Roast vegetables in the preheated oven for 20-25 minutes, stirring halfway through, until tender and slightly caramelized.

6. Divide cooked quinoa among serving bowls and top with roasted vegetables.

7. If desired, sprinkle with crumbled feta cheese and chopped fresh herbs, and drizzle with balsamic glaze.

8. Serve hot as a nourishing and flavorful meal.

58.Chocolate Banana Chia Seed Pudding

Ingredients:

- 2 ripe bananas
- 1/4 cup cocoa powder
- 2 tablespoons honey or maple syrup
- 1 teaspoon vanilla extract
- 1/2 cup chia seeds
- 2 cups milk of choice (such as almond milk, coconut milk)
- Optional toppings: sliced bananas, chopped nuts, shredded coconut

Instructions:

1. In a blender, combine ripe bananas, cocoa powder, honey or maple syrup, and vanilla extract. Blend until smooth.

2. Transfer the banana-chocolate mixture to a bowl and stir in chia seeds and milk.

3. Cover the bowl and refrigerate for at least 4 hours, or overnight, until the chia seeds have absorbed the liquid and the mixture has thickened into a pudding-like consistency.

4. Serve the chocolate banana chia seed pudding cold, topped with sliced bananas, chopped nuts, and shredded coconut if desired.

59.Turkey and Spinach Meatballs

Ingredients:

- 1 pound ground turkey

- 1 cup chopped spinach

- 1/4 cup grated Parmesan cheese

- 1/4 cup breadcrumbs

- 1 egg, beaten

- 2 cloves garlic, minced

- 1 teaspoon dried oregano

- 1 teaspoon dried basil

- Salt and pepper to taste

- Olive oil for cooking

Instructions:

1. Preheat your oven to 375°F (190°C) and line a baking sheet with parchment paper.

2. In a large mixing bowl, combine ground turkey, chopped spinach, grated Parmesan cheese,

breadcrumbs, beaten egg, minced garlic, dried oregano, dried basil, salt, and pepper.

3. Mix all ingredients until well combined.

4. Shape the mixture into meatballs, using about 1 tablespoon of the mixture for each meatball.

5. Place the meatballs on the prepared baking sheet.

6. Drizzle olive oil over the meatballs and bake in the preheated oven for 20-25 minutes, or until cooked through and lightly browned.

7. Serve the turkey and spinach meatballs hot with your favorite sauce or alongside pasta or salad.

60.Coconut Curry Vegetable Stir-Fry

Ingredients:

- 2 tablespoons coconut oil
- 1 onion, thinly sliced
- 2 cloves garlic, minced
- 1 tablespoon grated ginger
- 1 bell pepper, thinly sliced
- 1 cup broccoli florets
- 1 carrot, julienned
- 1 zucchini, sliced
- 1 can (14 ounces) coconut milk
- 2 tablespoons red curry paste
- 1 tablespoon soy sauce
- 1 tablespoon lime juice
- Salt and pepper to taste
- Cooked rice for serving
- Optional garnish: chopped cilantro, sliced green onions, lime wedges

Instructions:

1. Heat coconut oil in a large skillet or wok over medium-high heat.

2. Add thinly sliced onion, minced garlic, and grated ginger to the skillet. Sauté for 2-3 minutes until fragrant.

3. Add thinly sliced bell pepper, broccoli florets, julienned carrot, and sliced zucchini to the skillet. Stir-fry for 4-5 minutes until vegetables are tender-crisp.

4. In a small bowl, whisk together coconut milk, red curry paste, soy sauce, and lime juice.

5. Pour the coconut milk mixture over the vegetables in the skillet. Stir to coat evenly.

6. Cook for an additional 2-3 minutes until the sauce is heated through and the vegetables are well coated.

7. Season with salt and pepper to taste.

8. Serve the coconut curry vegetable stir-fry hot over cooked rice.

9. Garnish with chopped cilantro, sliced green onions, and lime wedges if desired.

61.Blueberry Oatmeal Muffins

Ingredients:

- 1 cup old-fashioned rolled oats

- 1 cup milk (any kind)

- 1 cup all-purpose flour

- 1/2 cup brown sugar

- 1 teaspoon baking powder

- 1/2 teaspoon baking soda

- 1/2 teaspoon salt

- 1/4 cup unsweetened applesauce

- 1/4 cup vegetable oil

- 1 egg

- 1 teaspoon vanilla extract

- 1 cup fresh or frozen blueberries

Instructions:

1. Preheat your oven to 375°F (190°C). Line a muffin tin with paper liners or grease the muffin cups.

2. In a bowl, combine rolled oats and milk. Let the mixture sit for 5-10 minutes to soften the oats.

3. In a separate large mixing bowl, whisk together all-purpose flour, brown sugar, baking powder, baking soda, and salt.

4. Add unsweetened applesauce, vegetable oil, egg, and vanilla extract to the oat and milk mixture. Stir until well combined.

5. Pour the wet ingredients into the dry ingredients and mix until just combined. Do not overmix.

6. Gently fold in fresh or frozen blueberries.

7. Divide the batter evenly among the prepared muffin cups, filling each about 3/4 full.

8. Bake in the preheated oven for 18-20 minutes, or until a toothpick inserted into the center of a muffin comes out clean.

9. Remove the muffins from the oven and let them cool in the muffin tin for 5 minutes before transferring to a wire rack to cool completely.

10. Enjoy the blueberry oatmeal muffins as a wholesome and delicious snack or breakfast option.

62. Vegetable Lentil Soup

Ingredients:

- 1 cup dried green or brown lentils, rinsed
- 4 cups vegetable broth
- 1 onion, diced
- 2 carrots, diced
- 2 celery stalks, diced
- 2 cloves garlic, minced
- 1 can (14 ounces) diced tomatoes
- 1 teaspoon dried thyme
- 1 teaspoon dried oregano
- Salt and pepper to taste
- 2 tablespoons olive oil
- Fresh parsley for garnish

Instructions:

1. In a large pot, heat olive oil over medium heat. Add diced onion, carrots, and celery. Sauté until vegetables are softened, about 5 minutes.

2. Add minced garlic to the pot and cook for another minute until fragrant.

3. Stir in rinsed lentils, vegetable broth, diced tomatoes with their juices, dried thyme, and dried oregano.

4. Bring the soup to a boil, then reduce heat to low and let it simmer for about 25-30 minutes, or until lentils are tender.

5. Season with salt and pepper to taste.

6. Serve hot, garnished with fresh parsley.

63.Honey Mustard Glazed Salmon

Ingredients:

- 4 salmon fillets

- Salt and pepper to taste

- 3 tablespoons Dijon mustard

- 2 tablespoons honey

- 1 tablespoon olive oil

- 1 tablespoon soy sauce

- 1 clove garlic, minced

- Optional garnish: chopped fresh dill

Instructions:

1. Preheat your oven to 400°F (200°C). Line a baking sheet with parchment paper.

2. Season salmon fillets with salt and pepper on both sides and place them on the prepared baking sheet.

3. In a small bowl, whisk together Dijon mustard, honey, olive oil, soy sauce, and minced garlic.

4. Brush the honey mustard glaze over the salmon fillets, coating them evenly.

5. Bake in the preheated oven for 12-15 minutes, or until salmon is cooked through and flakes easily with a fork.

6. Remove from the oven and garnish with chopped fresh dill if desired.

7. Serve hot with your favorite side dishes.

64. Mango Avocado Quinoa Salad

Ingredients:

- 1 cup quinoa, rinsed
- 2 cups water or vegetable broth
- 1 ripe mango, peeled and diced
- 1 ripe avocado, peeled, pitted, and diced
- 1/4 cup red onion, finely chopped
- 1/4 cup chopped fresh cilantro
- Juice of 1 lime
- 2 tablespoons olive oil
- Salt and pepper to taste

Instructions:

1. In a saucepan, combine quinoa and water or vegetable broth. Bring to a boil, then reduce heat

to low, cover, and simmer for 15-20 minutes until quinoa is cooked and liquid is absorbed.

2. Fluff cooked quinoa with a fork and transfer it to a large mixing bowl.

3. Add diced mango, diced avocado, finely chopped red onion, chopped fresh cilantro, lime juice, and olive oil to the bowl.

4. Gently toss all ingredients together until well combined.

5. Season with salt and pepper to taste.

6. Serve the mango avocado quinoa salad chilled or at room temperature as a refreshing side dish or light meal.

65.Grilled Vegetable Salad

Ingredients:

- 2 zucchinis, sliced lengthwise
- 2 bell peppers, halved and seeds removed
- 1 red onion, sliced into rounds
- 1 cup cherry tomatoes
- 2 tablespoons olive oil
- Salt and pepper to taste

- 2 tablespoons balsamic vinegar
- 1 tablespoon honey
- 1 clove garlic, minced
- 1 teaspoon Dijon mustard
- Fresh basil leaves for garnish

Instructions:

1. Preheat your grill to medium-high heat.

2. Brush sliced zucchinis, bell peppers, red onion rounds, and cherry tomatoes with olive oil. Season with salt and pepper.

3. Grill the vegetables until tender and lightly charred, about 3-5 minutes per side for zucchini and bell peppers, and 2-3 minutes for cherry tomatoes and red onion rounds. Remove from the grill and let cool slightly.

4. In a small bowl, whisk together balsamic vinegar, honey, minced garlic, and Dijon mustard to make the dressing.

5. Arrange grilled vegetables on a serving platter. Drizzle with the prepared dressing.

6. Garnish with fresh basil leaves before serving. This grilled vegetable salad is delicious served warm or at room temperature.

66.Stuffed Bell Peppers

Ingredients:

- 4 large bell peppers, halved and seeds removed
- 1 cup cooked quinoa
- 1 can (15 ounces) black beans, drained and rinsed
- 1 cup corn kernels (fresh, canned, or frozen)
- 1 cup diced tomatoes
- 1 cup shredded cheddar cheese
- 1 teaspoon ground cumin
- 1 teaspoon chili powder
- Salt and pepper to taste
- Optional garnish: chopped fresh cilantro, sour cream

Instructions:

1. Preheat your oven to 375°F (190°C). Grease a baking dish with olive oil.

2. In a large mixing bowl, combine cooked quinoa, black beans, corn kernels, diced tomatoes, shredded cheddar cheese, ground cumin, chili powder, salt, and pepper.

3. Spoon the quinoa and black bean mixture into each bell pepper half, pressing down gently to fill.

4. Place stuffed bell peppers in the prepared baking dish.

5. Cover the dish with aluminum foil and bake in the preheated oven for 25-30 minutes, or until bell peppers are tender.

6. Remove the foil and bake for an additional 5 minutes to melt the cheese and lightly brown the tops.

7. Garnish with chopped fresh cilantro and a dollop of sour cream before serving. These stuffed bell peppers make a satisfying and nutritious meal.

67. Banana Walnut Bread

Ingredients:

- 2 ripe bananas, mashed
- 1/3 cup melted butter or coconut oil
- 1/2 cup honey or maple syrup
- 2 eggs
- 1 teaspoon vanilla extract
- 1 3/4 cups all-purpose flour
- 1 teaspoon baking soda
- 1/2 teaspoon ground cinnamon

- 1/4 teaspoon salt

- 1/2 cup chopped walnuts

Instructions:

1. Preheat your oven to 350°F (175°C). Grease a 9x5-inch loaf pan.

2. In a large mixing bowl, combine mashed bananas, melted butter or coconut oil, honey or maple syrup, eggs, and vanilla extract. Mix until well combined.

3. In a separate bowl, whisk together all-purpose flour, baking soda, ground cinnamon, and salt.

4. Gradually add the dry ingredients to the wet ingredients, stirring until just combined. Be careful not to overmix.

5. Fold in chopped walnuts.

6. Pour the batter into the prepared loaf pan.

7. Bake in the preheated oven for 55-60 minutes, or until a toothpick inserted into the center comes out clean.

8. Allow the banana walnut bread to cool in the pan for 10 minutes before transferring to a wire rack to cool completely. Slice and enjoy this moist and flavorful bread as a snack or breakfast option.

68.Mediterranean Quinoa Salad

Ingredients:

- 1 cup quinoa, rinsed
- 2 cups water or vegetable broth
- 1 cup cherry tomatoes, halved
- 1 cucumber, diced
- 1/4 cup diced red onion
- 1/4 cup chopped fresh parsley
- 1/4 cup chopped fresh mint
- 1/4 cup crumbled feta cheese
- 1/4 cup Kalamata olives, sliced
- Juice of 1 lemon
- 2 tablespoons extra virgin olive oil
- Salt and pepper to taste

Instructions:

1. In a saucepan, combine quinoa and water or vegetable broth. Bring to a boil, then reduce heat to low, cover, and simmer for 15-20 minutes until quinoa is cooked and liquid is absorbed.

2. Fluff cooked quinoa with a fork and transfer it to a large mixing bowl.

3. Add cherry tomatoes, diced cucumber, diced red onion, chopped fresh parsley, chopped fresh mint, crumbled feta cheese, and sliced Kalamata olives to the bowl.

4. In a small bowl, whisk together lemon juice and extra virgin olive oil. Pour the dressing over the quinoa salad.

5. Toss all ingredients together until well combined.

6. Season with salt and pepper to taste.

7. Serve the Mediterranean quinoa salad chilled or at room temperature as a refreshing and flavorful side dish or light meal.

69. Lemon Garlic Roasted Chicken Thighs

Ingredients:

- 6 bone-in, skin-on chicken thighs
- 3 cloves garlic, minced
- Zest and juice of 1 lemon
- 2 tablespoons olive oil
- 1 teaspoon dried thyme
- 1 teaspoon dried rosemary
- Salt and pepper to taste

- Fresh parsley for garnish

Instructions:

1. Preheat your oven to 400°F (200°C). Line a baking sheet with parchment paper.

2. In a small bowl, combine minced garlic, lemon zest, lemon juice, olive oil, dried thyme, dried rosemary, salt, and pepper to make the marinade.

3. Pat chicken thighs dry with paper towels and place them on the prepared baking sheet.

4. Brush the marinade over the chicken thighs, coating them evenly.

5. Roast in the preheated oven for 35-40 minutes, or until chicken is cooked through and skin is crispy and golden brown.

6. Remove from the oven and let the chicken thighs rest for a few minutes.

7. Garnish with fresh parsley before serving. These lemon garlic roasted chicken thighs are delicious served with roasted vegetables or a side salad.

70.Creamy Mushroom Risotto

Ingredients:

- 1 tablespoon olive oil

- 1 tablespoon butter

- 1 onion, finely chopped

- 2 cloves garlic, minced

- 8 ounces (225g) mushrooms, sliced

- 1 cup Arborio rice

- 1/2 cup dry white wine

- 4 cups vegetable broth, warmed

- 1/4 cup grated Parmesan cheese

- Salt and pepper to taste

- Fresh parsley for garnish

Instructions:

1. In a large skillet or saucepan, heat olive oil and butter over medium heat.

2. Add finely chopped onion and minced garlic to the skillet. Sauté for 2-3 minutes until softened.

3. Add sliced mushrooms to the skillet and cook for 5-7 minutes until they release their juices and start to brown.

4. Stir in Arborio rice and cook for 1-2 minutes until rice is lightly toasted.

5. Pour dry white wine into the skillet and cook, stirring constantly, until the wine is absorbed.

6. Gradually add warm vegetable broth to the skillet, 1/2 cup at a time, stirring frequently and allowing the rice to absorb the broth before adding more.

7. Continue adding broth and cooking the rice until it is creamy and tender, about 20-25 minutes in total.

8. Stir in grated Parmesan cheese and season with salt and pepper to taste.

9. Garnish with fresh parsley before serving. This creamy mushroom risotto makes a comforting and satisfying meal.

71.Caprese Salad

Ingredients:

- 2 large ripe tomatoes, sliced

- 1 ball fresh mozzarella cheese, sliced

- Fresh basil leaves

- Extra virgin olive oil

- Balsamic glaze

- Salt and pepper to taste

Instructions:

1. Arrange the sliced tomatoes and fresh mozzarella cheese on a serving platter, alternating them.

2. Place a basil leaf between each tomato and mozzarella slice.

3. Drizzle extra virgin olive oil over the salad.

4. Drizzle balsamic glaze over the salad in a zigzag pattern.

5. Season with salt and pepper to taste.

6. Serve the Caprese salad immediately as a light and refreshing appetizer or side dish.

72.Lentil and Vegetable Curry

Ingredients:

- 1 cup dried lentils, rinsed
- 4 cups vegetable broth
- 2 tablespoons olive oil
- 1 onion, diced
- 2 cloves garlic, minced
- 1 tablespoon grated ginger
- 1 tablespoon curry powder
- 1 teaspoon ground turmeric
- 1 teaspoon ground cumin
- 1 teaspoon ground coriander
- 1 can (14 ounces) diced tomatoes
- 2 cups chopped mixed vegetables (such as carrots, bell peppers, zucchini)
- Salt and pepper to taste
- Cooked rice for serving
- Optional garnish: chopped fresh cilantro

Instructions:

1. In a large pot, heat olive oil over medium heat. Add diced onion and sauté until softened, about 5 minutes.

2. Add minced garlic and grated ginger to the pot. Cook for another minute until fragrant.

3. Stir in curry powder, ground turmeric, ground cumin, and ground coriander. Cook for 1-2 minutes until spices are toasted and fragrant.

4. Add rinsed lentils, vegetable broth, diced tomatoes with their juices, and chopped mixed vegetables to the pot.

5. Bring the curry to a boil, then reduce heat to low and let it simmer for about 20-25 minutes, or until lentils and vegetables are tender.

6. Season with salt and pepper to taste.

7. Serve the lentil and vegetable curry hot over cooked rice.

8. Garnish with chopped fresh cilantro if desired. This hearty and flavorful curry is perfect for a nourishing meal.

73.Spinach and Feta Stuffed Chicken Breast

Ingredients:

- 4 boneless, skinless chicken breasts
- Salt and pepper to taste
- 1 cup chopped spinach
- 1/2 cup crumbled feta cheese
- 2 tablespoons olive oil
- 2 cloves garlic, minced
- 1 teaspoon dried oregano
- 1 teaspoon dried thyme
- Juice of 1 lemon

Instructions:

1. Preheat your oven to 400°F (200°C).
2. Using a sharp knife, cut a pocket into each chicken breast.
3. Season the inside of each pocket with salt and pepper.
4. In a bowl, combine chopped spinach and crumbled feta cheese. Stuff each chicken breast with the spinach and feta mixture.

5. In a small bowl, whisk together olive oil, minced garlic, dried oregano, dried thyme, and lemon juice.

6. Brush the seasoned olive oil mixture over the stuffed chicken breasts.

7. Place the stuffed chicken breasts in a baking dish.

8. Bake in the preheated oven for 25-30 minutes, or until chicken is cooked through and juices run clear.

9. Serve the spinach and feta stuffed chicken breasts hot, accompanied by your favorite side dishes. Enjoy the flavorful combination of spinach, feta, and tender chicken.

74.Mango Coconut Smoothie

Ingredients:

- 1 ripe mango, peeled and diced

- 1/2 cup coconut milk

- 1/2 cup plain Greek yogurt

- 1 tablespoon honey or maple syrup (optional, depending on sweetness of mango)

- 1/2 teaspoon vanilla extract

- Ice cubes (optional)

Instructions:

1. Place diced mango, coconut milk, Greek yogurt, honey or maple syrup (if using), and vanilla extract in a blender.

2. Blend until smooth and creamy.

3. If desired, add ice cubes to the blender and blend until smooth.

4. Pour the mango coconut smoothie into glasses and serve immediately. Enjoy this refreshing and tropical beverage as a nutritious snack or breakfast option.

75.Stuffed Portobello Mushrooms

Ingredients:

- 4 large portobello mushrooms, stems removed

- 2 tablespoons olive oil

- 2 cloves garlic, minced

- 1/2 cup diced red bell pepper

- 1/2 cup diced zucchini

- 1/2 cup diced eggplant

- 1/4 cup chopped fresh parsley

- Salt and pepper to taste

- 1/2 cup shredded mozzarella cheese

Instructions:

1. Preheat your oven to 375°F (190°C).

2. Place portobello mushrooms on a baking sheet lined with parchment paper.

3. In a skillet, heat olive oil over medium heat. Add minced garlic and sauté for 1 minute until fragrant.

4. Add diced red bell pepper, diced zucchini, and diced eggplant to the skillet. Cook for 5-7 minutes until vegetables are tender.

5. Stir in chopped fresh parsley and season with salt and pepper to taste.

6. Spoon the vegetable mixture into the hollowed-out portobello mushrooms, dividing evenly.

7. Top each stuffed mushroom with shredded mozzarella cheese.

8. Bake in the preheated oven for 15-20 minutes, or until mushrooms are tender and cheese is melted and bubbly.

9. Serve the stuffed portobello mushrooms hot as a flavorful and satisfying appetizer or side dish.

76. Turkey and Vegetable Stir-Fry

Ingredients:

- 1 tablespoon vegetable oil
- 1 pound ground turkey
- 1 onion, thinly sliced
- 2 cloves garlic, minced
- 1 bell pepper, thinly sliced
- 1 cup broccoli florets
- 1 carrot, julienned
- 1/2 cup snap peas
- 1/4 cup soy sauce

- 2 tablespoons hoisin sauce

- 1 tablespoon rice vinegar

- Cooked rice for serving

- Optional garnish: sliced green onions, sesame seeds

Instructions:

1. Heat vegetable oil in a large skillet or wok over medium-high heat.

2. Add ground turkey to the skillet and cook, breaking it apart with a spoon, until browned and cooked through.

3. Add thinly sliced onion and minced garlic to the skillet. Sauté for 2-3 minutes until softened.

4. Add thinly sliced bell pepper, broccoli florets, julienned carrot, and snap peas to the skillet. Stir-fry for 4-5 minutes until vegetables are tender-crisp.

5. In a small bowl, whisk together soy sauce, hoisin sauce, and rice vinegar. Pour the sauce over the turkey and vegetables in the skillet.

6. Cook for an additional 2-3 minutes, stirring constantly, until the sauce is heated through and the ingredients are well coated.

7. Serve the turkey and vegetable stir-fry hot over cooked rice.

8. Garnish with sliced green onions and sesame seeds if desired. Enjoy this flavorful and nutritious stir-fry as a wholesome meal.

77.Sweet Potato and Black Bean Tacos

Ingredients:

- 2 medium sweet potatoes, peeled and diced
- 1 tablespoon olive oil
- 1 teaspoon chili powder
- 1/2 teaspoon ground cumin
- Salt and pepper to taste
- 1 can (15 ounces) black beans, drained and rinsed
- 8 small corn tortillas
- Toppings: sliced avocado, shredded lettuce, diced tomatoes, salsa, Greek yogurt or sour cream, lime wedges

Instructions:

1. Preheat your oven to 400°F (200°C). Line a baking sheet with parchment paper.

2. In a bowl, toss diced sweet potatoes with olive oil, chili powder, ground cumin, salt, and pepper until evenly coated.

3. Spread the seasoned sweet potatoes in a single layer on the prepared baking sheet.

4. Roast in the preheated oven for 20-25 minutes, or until sweet potatoes are tender and lightly browned.

5. Warm corn tortillas according to package instructions.

6. Assemble tacos by filling each tortilla with roasted sweet potatoes and black beans.

7. Top with sliced avocado, shredded lettuce, diced tomatoes, salsa, Greek yogurt or sour cream, and a squeeze of lime juice.

8. Serve the sweet potato and black bean tacos immediately as a delicious and satisfying meal.

78.Greek Yogurt Parfait

Ingredients:

- 1 cup Greek yogurt (plain or flavored)

- 1/2 cup granola

- 1/2 cup mixed fresh berries (such as strawberries, blueberries, raspberries)

- Honey or maple syrup (optional, for drizzling)

- Optional add-ins: sliced bananas, chopped nuts, shredded coconut

Instructions:

1. In a glass or bowl, layer Greek yogurt, granola, and mixed fresh berries.

2. Repeat the layers until the glass or bowl is filled.

3. Drizzle honey or maple syrup over the top if desired.

4. Garnish with optional add-ins such as sliced bananas, chopped nuts, or shredded coconut.

5. Serve the Greek yogurt parfait immediately as a nutritious and delicious breakfast or snack option.

79.Teriyaki Salmon with Vegetable Stir-Fry

Ingredients:

- 4 salmon fillets

- Salt and pepper to taste

- 1 tablespoon olive oil

- 1/4 cup teriyaki sauce

- 2 cups mixed vegetables (such as bell peppers, broccoli, snap peas, carrots), sliced or julienned

- Cooked rice for serving

- Optional garnish: sliced green onions, sesame seeds

Instructions:

1. Season salmon fillets with salt and pepper to taste.

2. Heat olive oil in a skillet over medium-high heat. Add salmon fillets to the skillet and cook for 3-4 minutes on each side, or until salmon is cooked through and flakes easily with a fork.

3. Brush teriyaki sauce over the cooked salmon fillets.

4. In the same skillet, add mixed vegetables and stir-fry for 4-5 minutes until vegetables are tender-crisp.

5. Serve the teriyaki salmon hot over cooked rice, accompanied by the vegetable stir-fry.

6. Garnish with sliced green onions and sesame seeds if desired. Enjoy this flavorful and nutritious dish as a wholesome meal.

80.Vegetable Frittata

Ingredients:

- 8 large eggs
- 1/4 cup milk or cream
- Salt and pepper to taste
- 2 tablespoons olive oil
- 1 small onion, diced
- 1 bell pepper, diced
- 1 cup sliced mushrooms
- 1 cup spinach leaves
- 1/2 cup grated cheese (such as cheddar or feta)
- Fresh herbs for garnish (such as parsley or chives)

Instructions:

1. Preheat your oven to 375°F (190°C).

2. In a large mixing bowl, whisk together eggs, milk or cream, salt, and pepper until well combined. Set aside.

3. Heat olive oil in a large oven-safe skillet over medium heat. Add diced onion and cook until softened, about 2-3 minutes.

4. Add diced bell pepper and sliced mushrooms to the skillet. Cook for another 3-4 minutes until vegetables are tender.

5. Add spinach leaves to the skillet and cook until wilted.

6. Pour the egg mixture evenly over the vegetables in the skillet.

7. Sprinkle grated cheese over the top.

8. Transfer the skillet to the preheated oven and bake for 15-20 minutes, or until the frittata is set and the top is golden brown.

9. Remove from the oven and let the frittata cool for a few minutes before slicing.

10. Garnish with fresh herbs before serving. This vegetable frittata makes a delicious and versatile meal for any time of day.

81.Honey Garlic Shrimp Stir-Fry

Ingredients:

- 1 pound large shrimp, peeled and deveined
- Salt and pepper to taste
- 2 tablespoons olive oil
- 3 cloves garlic, minced
- 1 tablespoon grated ginger
- 1 bell pepper, thinly sliced
- 1 cup broccoli florets
- 1/4 cup soy sauce
- 2 tablespoons honey
- Cooked rice or noodles for serving
- Optional garnish: sliced green onions, sesame seeds

Instructions:

1. Season shrimp with salt and pepper to taste.

2. Heat olive oil in a large skillet or wok over medium-high heat. Add minced garlic and grated ginger to the skillet. Cook for 1 minute until fragrant.

3. Add shrimp to the skillet and cook for 2-3 minutes on each side until pink and opaque. Remove shrimp from the skillet and set aside.

4. In the same skillet, add thinly sliced bell pepper and broccoli florets. Stir-fry for 3-4 minutes until vegetables are tender-crisp.

5. In a small bowl, whisk together soy sauce and honey. Pour the sauce over the vegetables in the skillet.

6. Return cooked shrimp to the skillet and toss everything together until well coated in the sauce.

7. Cook for another minute until heated through.

8. Serve the honey garlic shrimp stir-fry hot over cooked rice or noodles.

9. Garnish with sliced green onions and sesame seeds if desired. Enjoy this flavorful and easy-to-make dish as a quick meal option.

== THE END ==

Thank you for choosing our book! We trust that it met or exceeded your expectations.

If you enjoyed our book, kindly consider sharing your thoughts in a review on social media. Your feedback is invaluable as it aids us in enhancing our products and services for future readers.

We sincerely appreciate your support and extend our best wishes to you.